# ESSENTIAL STAPLE FOODS FOR A GOOD DIET

IMPROVE YOUR HEALTH WITH THE NUTRIENTS
YOUR BODY REALLY NEEDS, PROTEINS,
CARBOHYDRATES, FATS

Jessy M. Brown

# Table of Contents

# INTRODUCTION

Healthy eating is not about rigid doctrines of nutrition, being unrealistically skinny or depriving yourself of the food you love. Instead, it's about feeling great, being more vigorous and staying as healthy as possible, all of which can be accomplished by learning some basic nutrition concepts and using them in a way that works for you.

Healthy eating begins with learning how to "eat smart," not just what you eat, but how you eat. Your food choices can reduce your risk of diseases such as heart disease, cancer, and diabetes, as well as fight depression.

In addition, learning smart eating habits can increase your energy, increase your memory, and stabilize your mood. You can expand your range of healthy food choices and learn to plan ahead to produce and maintain a rewarding and intelligent diet.

# CHAPTER I:
# BECOME SMARTER

Instead of worrying too much about counting calories or evaluating portion sizes, consider your diet in terms of color, variety, and freshness; then it should be easier to make healthy choices. Focus on discovering the foods you like and simple recipes that incorporate a couple of fresh ingredients. Little by little, your diet will become healthier and more delicious.

Cooking with easy ingredients brings you back to the basic food ingredients, the way Grandma used to cook them. By using simple ingredients in your meal recipes, you can limit or eliminate the negative effect of processed and chemical-laden foods on you and your loved ones.

Healthy cooking with easy ingredients

requires a little advance planning to organize your kitchen. We lead busy lives today, so the last thing we want to do is add more time to our busy schedules, that's why you need to plan on making your kitchen more efficient and reducing your shopping time.

One of the first things you will want to accomplish is to look through your kitchen and study all of your food labels, once you get to foods that are healthy for you you might want to make a list of what you will need to complete the work of remodeling your kitchen.

With easy-to-handle basic ingredients, you can quickly make a variety of different foods that are fast and healthy.

*There are many basic foods you can store in your pantry*

- ✓ Whole grains
- ✓ Dried beans
- ✓ Natural sweeteners
- ✓ Beneficial oils and good fats

✓ Dried spices

*There are many basic foods you can store in your freezer*

✓ Vegetables
✓ Fruits and berries
✓ Meats and broths
✓ Cheese

Start slowly and make changes in your eating habits over time.

Trying to make your diet healthy overnight is neither realistic nor bright. Altering everything at once commonly leads to cheating or abandoning your fresh food plan.

Take small steps, such as adding a salad (full of colorful vegetables) to your diet once a day or switching from butter to olive oil while cooking. As your small changes become a habit, you can continue to add more healthy choices to your diet.

Every alteration you make to improve your diet is important. You don't have to be perfect and you don't have to totally eliminate the foods you enjoy to have a smart diet. The long-term goal is to feel good, have more energy, and decrease the risk of cancer and disease. Don't let your stumbles disrupt you - every healthy food choice you make is important.

### Consider water and exercise

- **Water**

Water helps eliminate waste and toxins from our systems. However, many people due to dehydration feel a lot of fatigue, low energy and headaches. It is common to confuse thirst with hunger, so staying well hydrated will also help you make smarter food choices.

- **Physical activity**

Find something active you like to do and add it to your day, just as you would add healthy vegetables, cranberries or salmon. The benefits of lifelong physical activity are plentiful, and regular exercise can even motivate you to make healthy food choices a habit.

# CHAPTER II:
# HOW TO MAINTAIN A
# BALANCE IN THE DIET?

People much of the time think that smart eating is an all-or-nothing proposition, but one of the main bases of any healthy diet is moderation. Despite what fad diets make you think, we all need a balance of carbohydrates, proteins, fats, fibers, vitamins and minerals to maintain a healthy body.

If you ban certain foods or food groups, it is natural to want those foods more and then feel like a loser if you give in to temptation.

If you are attracted to sweet, salty, or unhealthy foods, start by reducing portion sizes and not eating them as often. Later you may find yourself yearning for them less or thinking of them as occasional indulgences.

Healthy foods are crucial to maintaining a healthy diet and lifestyle. Times have changed and there are many nutritious food choices available.

- **Remember the Food Pyramid?**

The old USDA food pyramid has changed. We always recognized it as the 6 basic food groups. It has been retrofitted and now has 5 basic groups that include whole grains, seeds, nuts, and vegetable oils.

### Fats, Oils and Sweets

✓ Healthy sources of fat are nuts, fish, and vegetable oils.

✓ Reduce margarine, butter, lard, and foods that

contain them. This reduces solid fats.

✓ Use sodium, trans fats, and saturated fats sparingly.

✓ Unsaturated oils such as olive or sunflower oil should be used.

✓ Meat, Poultry, Fish, Eggs, Dried Beans and Nuts

✓ Use lean cuts of meat.

✓ Choose more fish, beans, peas, nuts, and seeds.

Based on a 2000 calorie diet, you would eat 5 1/2 ounces a day.

## Milk, yogurt, cheese and dairy products

Choose low-fat assortments such as skim milk, low-fat buttermilk, yogurt, and low-fat cheeses. Tofu and soy are first-class options.

Based on a 2000 calorie diet, you would consume 3 cups daily.

### *Fruit*

✓ You are able to use all kinds of fruits. They can be frozen, dry and fresh.

✓ Fruits are low in fat, contain fiber, minerals and vitamins. They also help curb the taste for sweets!

Based on a 2000 calorie diet, you would eat 2 cups of fruit a day.

### *Vegetables*

Choose more dark green leafy vegetables such as broccoli and spinach.

✓ Choose sweet potatoes, carrots, and other vegetables.

✓ Remove peas and dried beans such as lentils and kidney beans or pinto beans.

Based on a 2000 calorie diet you would consume 2 and a half cups each day.

### *Grain*

✓ Choose whole grains, breads, crackers, rice, or pasta. Eat a minimum of 3 ounces daily. These are loaded with complex carbohydrates and fiber.

✓ A slice of bread is about one ounce, 1 bowl (about one cup) of breakfast cereal, 1/2 bagel or English muffin, 1/2 cup of pasta, or rice.

Based on a 2000 calorie diet, you would eat 6 ounces daily.

It is crucial that you choose healthy foods from each group to get the nutrients your body requires.

- ***Think of smaller portions.***

Portion sizes have increased lately, especially in restaurants. When eating out, choose a starter instead of a main course, share a dish with a friend, and don't order anything large. At home, use smaller dishes, consider portion sizes in realistic terms, and start with little.

Visual cues can help with portion size; your serving of meat, fish, or chicken should be the size of a deck of cards. A teaspoon of oil or dressing is about the size of a matchbox and your slice of bread should be the size of a CD box.

# CHAPTER III:
# THE KEY IS AT
# BREAKFAST.

Eat with others whenever possible. Eating with others has countless social and emotional advantages, especially for children, and allows you to model healthy eating habits. Eating in front of the TV or computer often leads to senseless overeating.

Chew your food slowly, savoring each bite. We tend to rush through our meals, really forgetting to taste the flavors and feel the textures of what's in our mouths. Reconnect with the pleasure of eating.

Ask yourself if you're really hungry, or drink a glass of water to see if you're thirsty instead of hungry. During a meal, stop eating before you feel full. It actually takes a few minutes for the brain to tell your body that you've had an adequate diet, so eat slowly.

- **Breakfast and eat lighter meals throughout the day.**

A healthy breakfast can boost your metabolism, and eating small, healthy meals throughout the day (instead of the standard three large meals) keeps your energy and metabolism on track.

Breakfast is really important in any weight loss program. A fit breakfast is really the most crucial meal of the day.

*A well-balanced, nutritious morning meal keeps your energy levels at their peak.*

**- Increase your efforts to lose weight.** Research shows that people who eat breakfast are more successful at losing weight and maintaining that weight loss.

*- Sharpen your brain.* Fit breakfast eaters will be more alert than those who start the day with a high-fat meal.

*- Protect your circulatory system.* One study found that people who ate breakfast with high-quality protein and good quality carbohydrate, rather than refined cereals, had a lower risk of heart disease.

*- Boost your immune system, burn fat and add muscle.* A fit breakfast will help you start the day with essential nutrients to add lean muscle, burn fat and recover from those intense exercises, as well as strengthen your immune system and keep it free of disease.

Eating anything you want for breakfast will not give you the wellness benefits mentioned above. Skipping breakfast or eating unhealthy foods can make you age much faster. Eating a good healthy breakfast will improve your health, improve your body, improve your quality of life and add years to your life.

- **_Healthy Breakfast Foods_**

**_Rolled oats, flaxseed, blueberries and almonds._** For me, this is an incredible breakfast. Flake oats are probably the healthiest choice, but if you're in a hurry, the instant type of oatmeal will be fine (it doesn't have as much fiber, but the extra ingredients make up for it).

After bombarding the oats, add the ground flaxseed, frozen blueberries and sliced almonds. You can add a little cinnamon and honey (not much) if you are using oatmeal flakes. Those are 4 powerful foods, full of fiber, nutrients, proteins and healthy fats, with only a few minutes of preparation. And very tasty!

Any high-fiber whole grain cereal is a good choice. Put on low-fat milk or soy milk, maybe some berries if you want.

**_Scrambled tofu._** Healthier than

scrambled eggs. Put a few onions, green peppers or other vegetables, a little light soy sauce or tamari, perhaps a little garlic powder, and black pepper, sauté with a little olive oil. Eat with whole wheat toast. Fast and delicious.

**Fresh berries, yogurt and granola.** Get low-fat yogurt or soy yogurt; pick a few extra berries or fruits, and add a healthy cereal.

**Grapefruit with whole wheat toast and almond butter.** Add a little sugar on top of the grapefruit. Almond butter is better for you than peanut butter, because it contains many proteins that keep you satiated.

**Fresh fruit salad.** Chop some apples, melons, berries, oranges, pears, bananas, grapes.... or whatever your favorite fruits are. Add a little lemon or lemon juice.

**Protein shake.** Use soy protein powder, but but buttermilk also works well. Mix with low-fat milk or soy milk, some frozen blueberries, and perhaps a little almond butter or oatmeal. That may sound weird, but it's really cool, and a nice stuffing. A little ground flax seed also works well.

***Eggs with peppers.*** Egg whites are healthier than egg yolks. Stir in a little olive oil, red and green peppers, perhaps broccoli, onions and black pepper. You can combine it with whole wheat toast.

***Cottage cheese and fruit.*** Get low-fat cottage cheese. Add any kind of fruit. Apples, citrus fruits, berries, etc. Mix and enjoy!

- ***Eat fruits and vegetables of all colors***

Eat a rainbow of fruits and vegetables every day, the brighter the better. Fruits and vegetables are the basis of a healthy diet: they are low in calories and dense in nutrients, which means they are packed with vitamins, minerals, antioxidants and fiber.

Fruits and vegetables should be part of every meal and your first choice for a snack - aim for a lower limit of 5 servings per day. The antioxidants and extra nutrients in fruits and vegetables help protect against particular types of cancer and other diseases.

Brighter, deeper colored fruits and vegetables have higher concentrations of vitamins, minerals and antioxidants, and assorted colors provide a variety of benefits. Some excellent options are:

- *Green vegetables:*

Vegetables are filled with calcium, magnesium, iron, potassium, zinc, vitamins A, C, E, and K, and help strengthen the blood and respiratory systems. Be adventurous with your vegetables and diversify beyond shiny, dark green lettuce; kale, mustard greens, broccoli, Chinese cabbage are just a couple of options.

- *Sweet vegetables:*

Naturally, sweet vegetables bring healthy sweetness to your meals and reduce your cravings for extra sweets. Examples of sweet vegetables include corn, carrots, beets, sweet potatoes, winter squash, and onions.

- **Fruits:**

A wide assortment of fruits is equally vital for a healthy diet. The fruit provides fibre, vitamins and antioxidants. Berries fight cancer, apples provide fiber, oranges and mangoes provide vitamin C, and so on.

Don't forget to buy fresh and local produce if possible.

# CHAPTER IV: CARBOHYDRATES AND WHOLE GRAINS

Choose healthy carbohydrates and fiber sources, particularly whole grains, for long-lasting energy. In addition to being delicious and enjoyable, whole grains are rich in photochemicals and antioxidants, which help protect against coronary heart disease, especially cancer and diabetes. Studies have shown that people who eat more whole grains tend to have a healthier heart.

*Healthy carbohydrates* (occasionally known as good carbohydrates) include whole grains, beans, fruits, and vegetables. Healthy carbohydrates are digested slowly, helping you feel fuller longer and keeping blood glucose and insulin levels stable.

**Unhealthy** (or bad) **carbohydrates** are foods such as white flour, refined sugar, and white rice that have been stripped of all bran, fiber, and nutrients. Unhealthy carbohydrates are quickly digested and cause spikes in blood glucose and energy levels.

- ### *How to consume more healthy carbohydrates?*

Include an assortment of whole grains in your healthy diet, including whole wheat, brown rice, millet, quinoa, and barley. Try different grains to discover your favorites.

Make sure you're really getting whole grains. Note that the words ground stone, multigrain, 100% wheat, or bran can be deceptive. Look for the words "whole grain" or "100% whole wheat" at the top of the ingredient list. In the United States, check for whole grain seals that differentiate between partial whole grains and 100% whole grains.

*Stay away from:* Refined foods such as breads, pastas, and breakfast cereals that are not whole grains.

### ❖ *Whole Grain Italian Bread Salad Recipe*

This Italian peasant dish is nothing but hard bread, tomatoes and olive oil, but I like to add something crunchy and green. It's also a good vehicle for leftover grilled vegetables, such as eggplants, mushrooms or courgettes, or for hard-boiled eggs or anchovies. If tomatoes are not in season, try the dried fruit version below.

- ✓ 8 ounces whole grain bread (4 thick slices)
- ✓ 4 stalks celery or 1 small fennel bulb, thinly sliced
- ✓ 1/4 cup olive oil
- ✓ 2 tablespoons balsamic vinegar
- ✓ 1 1/2 pounds ripe tomatoes, seeded and chopped

- ✓ 1/2 red onion, thinly sliced
- ✓ Salt and black pepper
- ✓ 1/2 cup chopped fresh basil

## Preparation

Heat oven to 400 F. Place bread on a baking and roasting tray, turning once or twice, until golden brown and dry, about 10-20 minutes, depending on the thickness of the slices. Remove from oven and cool.

Place celery, oil, vinegar, tomatoes and onion in a large salad bowl. Sprinkle with salt and lots of pepper and stir.

Fill a large bowl with tap water and soak the bread for about 3 minutes. Gently squeeze the slices until they are dry, then crumble them into the salad bowl. Mix well and let stand for 15 to 20 minutes (or up to one hour). Just before serving, taste, adjust seasoning if necessary and mix with basil.

### ❖ *Whole-grain bread salad with dried fruit*

Remove the tomatoes and basil and replace the onion with 2 medium shallots.

In Step 2, mix celery or fennel and dress with 1 cup chopped dried fruit (figs, dates, apricots, cherries, cranberries or raisins are all good) and 1 tablespoon chopped fresh sage.

Garnish with toasted hazelnuts or almonds.

# CHAPTER V: DIFFERENCE BETWEEN GOOD FATS AND BAD FATS

Large sources of healthy fats are required to nourish your brain, heart and cells, as well as your hair, skin and nails. Abundant foods, particularly omega-3 fats called EPA and DHA, are especially important and can reduce cardiovascular disease, improve your mood, and help prevent dementia.

For years, dietitians and doctors have preached the advantages of a low-fat diet. We've been told that reducing the amount of fat we eat is the key to losing weight, controlling cholesterol, and preventing health problems. But when it comes to your mental and physical health, simply "cutting the fat" is not enough.

Research shows that more than the sum total of fat in your diet, it's the types of fat you eat that really matter. Bad fats add to your cholesterol and your risk of particular diseases, while beneficial fats have the opposite effect, protecting your heart and defending your overall health. In fact, large fats - such as omega-3 fats - are absolutely essential not only for your physical health but also for your emotional well-being.

- **_Add healthy fats to your diet_**

- **_Monounsaturated fats:_** These are vegetable oils such as canola oil, peanut oil and olive oil, as well as avocados, walnuts, almonds, hazelnuts, etc; and seeds such as pumpkin seeds, sesame, chia, etc.

- **_Polyunsaturated Fats:_** These are the

Omega-3 and Omega-6 fatty acids found in fatty fish such as salmon, herring, mackerel, anchovies, sardines and some cold water fish oil supplements. Additional sources of polyunsaturated fats are unheated sunflower, corn, soybean, flaxseed, and nut oils.

- **Reduce or eliminate bad fats from your diet**

- **Saturated fats:** You are mainly found in animal sources, including red meat and whole milk dairy products.

- **Trans fats:** You are found in vegetable shorteners, some margarines, crackers and sweets, snacks, fried foods, baked goods, and additional processed foods made with partially hydrogenated vegetable oils.

When you focus on healthy fats, a good place to start is to reduce your intake of saturated fats. Saturated fats are found mainly in animal products such as red meat and whole milk dairy products.

Poultry and fish also contain saturated fat, but less than red meat. Additional sources of saturated fat include tropical vegetable oils such as coconut oil and palm oil.

- ***Easy ways to reduce saturated fat***
  - ✓ Eat less red meat (beef, pork, or lamb) and more fish and chicken.
  - ✓ Try to eat lean cuts of meat and stick to white meat, which has less saturated fat.
  - ✓ Bake or broil instead of frying.
  - ✓ Remove the skin from the chicken and remove as much fat as possible from the meat before cooking.
  - ✓ Stay away from meats, vegetables, empanadas, and fried foods.
  - ✓ Choose low-fat milk and low-fat cheeses such as

mozzarella if possible. Enjoy high-fat dairy products in moderation.

✓ Use liquid vegetable oils such as olive oil or canola oil instead of lard or butter.

A trans fat is a normal fat molecule that has been bent and deformed during a procedure called hydrogenation. During this procedure, the liquid vegetable oil is heated and mixed with hydrogen gas.

Partially hydrogenated vegetable oils make them more stable and less prone to spoilage, which is very good for food manufacturers, but very bad for you.

No amount of trans fat is good for you. Trans fats add up to major health problems, from heart disease to cancer.

- *Sources of trans fats*

Many people think of margarine when they imagine trans fats, and it's true that some margarines are full of them.

However, the main source of trans fats in the Western diet comes from commercially prepared baked goods and snacks:

*- Baked goods -* cookies, crackers, cakes, muffins, cake husks, pizza dough, and some breads such as buns for hamburgers.

*- Fried foods -* doughnuts, chips, fried chicken, chicken nuggets and hard tacos shells.

*- Appetizers - fries*, corn, and tortillas; sweets; popcorn packaged or in the microwave.

*- Solid fats -* stick margarine and semi-solid vegetable shortening

*- Premixed products -* cake mix, pancake mix and chocolate drink mix

While shopping, read the labels and look for "partially hydrogenated oil" on the components. Even if the food claims to be free of trans fats, this component makes it suspicious.

With margarine, choose the soft tub versions and make sure the product has zero grams of trans fat and does not contain partially hydrogenated oils.

When eating out, put fried foods, cookies, and other baked goods on your "skip" list. Stay away from these products unless you know the restaurant has removed trans fats from your food.

Stay away from fast food. Most states do not have fast food labeling ordinances, and may even advertise it as cholesterol-free when cooked in vegetable oil.

When you go out to dinner, ask your servant or person at the bar what type of oil your food will be cooked in. If it is partially hydrogenated oil, run in the opposite direction or ask if your food can be prepared using olive oil, which most restaurants have in stock.

Okay, then you realize that you have to

avoid saturated fats and trans fats... but how do you get the best for your monounsaturated and polyunsaturated fats that everybody keeps arguing about?

The most beneficial sources of healthy monounsaturated and polyunsaturated fats are vegetable oils, nuts, seeds and fish.

- *Cook with olive oil.* Use olive oil for cooking on the stove, instead of butter, stick margarine, or lard. For baking, try canola or vegetable oil.

- *Eat more avocados.* Try them on sandwiches or salads or make guacamole. In addition to being loaded with healthy fats for the heart and brain, they are a meal that fills and is enjoyable.

- *Grab the nuts.* You can also add nuts to vegetarian dishes or use them instead of bread crumbs in chicken or fish.

- *Aperitif with olives.* Olives are rich in monounsaturated fats. But unlike most other high-fat foods, they are a low-calorie snack if eaten alone. Try them simply or make a tapenade to get wet.

**- *Dress up your own salad.***
Commercial dressings are often high in saturated fats or made with trans fat oils. Produce your own healthy dressings with cold pressed olive oil, flaxseed oil, or high-quality sesame oil.

Good fat can become bad if heat, light, or oxygen damage it. Polyunsaturated fats are the most delicate. Oils rich in polyunsaturated fats (such as linseed oil) should be refrigerated and stored in an opaque container. Cooking with these oils also damages fats.

### • *Omega-3 fatty acids: superfats for the brain and heart*

Omega-3 fatty acids are a kind of polyunsaturated fat. While all types of monounsaturated and polyunsaturated fats are excellent for you, omega-3 fats are proving to be particularly beneficial.

We are still learning about the many advantages of omega-3 fatty acids, but research has shown that they can:

- ✓ Prevent and reduce the symptoms of depression
- ✓ Protect against memory loss and dementia
- ✓ Reduce the risk of heart disease, stroke, and cancer
- ✓ Relieve arthritis, joint pain, and inflammatory skin conditions
- ✓ Maintain a healthy pregnancy

Omega-3 fatty acids are very centered in the brain. Research shows that they play a vital role in cognitive function (memory, problem-solving ability, etc.) and also in emotional health.

Getting more omega-3 fatty acids in your diet can help you fight fatigue, sharpen your memory and balance your mood. Studies have shown that omega-3s may be helpful in the treatment of depression, attention deficit/hyperactivity disorder (ADHD), and manic depression.

There are many different types of omega-3 fatty acids such as fish: The most beneficial food source of omega-3s.

Omega-3 fats are a kind of essential fatty acid, which means they are essential for health, but your body can't produce them. You may only get omega-3 fatty acids from food.

The most beneficial sources are fatty fish such as salmon, herring, mackerel, anchovies or sardines, or supplements of high quality cold water fish oil. Canned albacore tuna and lake trout can also be great sources, depending on how the fish were raised and processed.

A few individuals avoid shellfish because they are concerned about mercury or other possible toxins in fish. However, most experts agree that the advantages of eating two servings a week of these cold water fatty fish are very beneficial.

If you are vegetarian or don't like fish, you can still get your omega-3 dose by eating algae (which are high in DHA) or a supplement of algae and chia oil capsules.

# CHAPTER VI:
# THE QUALITY OF
# PROTEINS

Proteins give us the energy to get up and move on. Food proteins are separated into the twenty amino acids that are the body's basic units for growth and energy, and are crucial for maintaining cells, tissues, and organs.

A lack of protein in our diet can slow growth, decrease muscle mass, decrease immunity, and weaken the heart and respiratory system.

Protein is especially crucial for young people, whose bodies grow and move daily.

Calcium is one of the key nutrients your

body needs to stay strong and healthy. It is an essential component of lifelong bone health in both men and women, among many other important functions.

*Here are some guidelines for including protein in your smart diet:*

Try a variety of protein types. Whether you're vegetarian or not, trying different sources of protein-such as beans, nuts, seeds, peas, tofu, and soy products-will open up new options for enjoying healthy meals.

> ✓ Soy products: Try tofu, soy milk, tempeh and veggie burgers for a change.
> ✓ Stay away from salted or sugary nuts and refried beans.
> ✓ Beans: Black beans, white beans, chickpeas and lentils are good choices.
> ✓ Nuts: Almonds, walnuts and pistachios are good choices.

Reduce the size of your protein portions.

Most individuals in the United States eat too much protein. Try to stay away from protein being the center of your food. It should focus on equal portions of protein, whole grains, and vegetables.

You should also eat quality protein sources, such as fresh fish, chicken or turkey, tofu, eggs, beans, or nuts. When you eat meat, chicken, or turkey, buy meat that does not contain hormones or antibiotics.

The bottom line is that it is crucial to pay attention to what comes with protein in your food choices. Vegetable sources of protein, such as beans, nuts, and whole grains, are excellent choices because they provide healthy fiber, vitamins, and minerals. Nuts are also an excellent source of healthy fats.

The best animal protein options are fish and poultry. If you like red meats, such as beef, pork or lamb, get the leanest cuts, choose moderate portions and make them just an occasional component of your diet, for several reasons.

There is substantial evidence that substituting fish, poultry, beans, or nuts for red meat may help prevent heart disease, and that reducing red meat may reduce the risk of diabetes.

Processed meats, in particular, have been more closely linked to cardiovascular disease and diabetes, at least in part because of their high sodium content.

You and your bones will benefit from eating lots of calcium-rich foods. It is advisable to consume a daily dose of magnesium and vitamins D and K (nutrients that help calcium to fulfill its function).

Suggested calcium levels are 1000 mg per day, 1200 mg if you are over fifty years of age. Take a supplement of vitamin D and calcium if you don't get the right nutrients in your diet.

- **These are the great sources of calcium:**
  -

  ✓ **Dairy:** Dairy products are abundant in calcium in a form that is easily digestible and absorbed by the body. Sources include milk, yogurt, and cheese.

  ✓ **Vegetables:** Many vegetables, especially leafy greens, are rich sources of calcium. Try turnip greens, mustard greens, cabbage leaves, kale, romaine lettuce, celery, broccoli, fennel, summer squash, green beans, Brussels sprouts, asparagus and crimini mushrooms.

  ✓ **Beans:** For a different source of calcium, try black beans, pinto beans, red beans, white beans, black-eyed beans, or baked beans.

# CONCLUSION

Healthy eating begins with excellent planning. You'll have won half the battle of a healthy diet if you have a well-equipped kitchen, lots of quick and simple recipes, and lots of healthy snacks.

- **_Get your meals per week or even per month_**

One of the best ways to have a healthy diet is to prepare your own food and eat regularly. Choose some healthy recipes that you and your loved ones like and establish a meal schedule around you.

If you eat cheaply, it is still crucial to consider the quality and purity of the food you buy. The way food is grown or bred influences its quality and also its health. Organically grown foods reduce potential health and environmental hazards from pesticides, irradiation and additives. An investment in your food today could save you money on your health bills later.

*Here are a couple of ways to save your money when you buy high quality organic food:*

Buy the best possible quality for the foods you eat the most. This way you reduce your exposure to things like pesticides, herbicides and antibiotics, while increasing the nutritional value of your foods. Organic foods have higher levels of antioxidants and several vitamins and minerals such as vitamin C, calcium, magnesium and iron.

Use food income savings to buy higher quality food. If conceivable, concentrate on purchasing sources of organic, grass-fed or free-access meat and dairy products because of the likely higher concentration of antibiotics and hormones that can be transmitted to you.

Teach yourself. When you understand

which product has the most chemical residues (and which has the least) you can choose to buy organic food or food from local farmers who do not use chemicals, and others grown conventionally.

Try cooking on weekends or one day a week, and make extra food to freeze or reserve for a special night. Cooking ahead saves time and money, and it's rewarding to know that you have a home-cooked meal waiting to be consumed.

Challenge yourself to prepare 2 or 3 dinners that can be prepared without having to go to the store, using things from your pantry, freezer and spice rack. A delicious wholemeal pasta dinner with a quick tomato sauce or a quick and easy black bean quesadilla on a wholemeal tortilla (among countless other recipes) can act as your favorite meal when you're simply too busy to shop or cook.

Eating healthy foods doesn't have to be

expensive. In fact, preparing your own meals can be a good way to help your family save money. Be original and have fun doing it!

- ***Some tips for saving money by preparing healthy foods:***

Replace vegetable protein with meat protein in some of your meals, particularly if you tend to eat meat at most meals. Legumes, particularly when bought in their dry form, cost much less than meat.

Discover a large agricultural market where local vegetables are sold. Frequently you can find amazing deals on really fresh produce. In addition, if you go toward the end of the market, sellers often sell what's left at even lower prices.

Buy wholesale. Find a grocery store that sells grains, legumes, nuts, seeds, and other bulk items. Store food in glass jars to keep it fresh.

Make your own version of items such as

salad dressing or smoothies. They'll be a lot healthier if you make yours and they're really simple.

*- Simple salad dressing:* olive oil, vinegar, mustard, herbs and a little salt and pepper.

*- Beat:* ½ banana, 6 strawberries, a handful of blueberries, liquid of your choice (i.e., some natural juice or low-fat milk) and blend until smooth.

*- Pack a lunch:* Bring leftovers or buy ingredients to make your own lunch. You'll save tons of money and be healthier for yourself.

*- A smart diet can include snacks:* Snacks can help keep our blood glucose level more even by giving us constant energy instead of the more common ups and downs in the energy level.

- **Smart snack ideas**

*Fruits and nuts -* This fantastic combination gives us fiber and protein for a nutritious snack. Eat a piece of fresh fruit and a handful of nuts. An excellent combination is the fruit with walnut butter spread on top.

**Yogurt parfait** - Low-fat natural yogurt with mixed fresh fruits. Using natural yogurt you decide how much sweetener to add. Likewise, try adding a touch of vanilla or cinnamon for different flavors. For a more satisfying snack, add a pinch of cereal or granola.

**Popcorn** - Make your own light popcorn for an excellent and tasty snack. You can even be adventurous with spices. Try adding curry, onion powder or anything else you like.

**Hummus and vegetables** - The chickpeas in hummus provide a lot of fiber and protein; it has no cholesterol and is a very satisfying and tasty snack.

*What if I just don't have time to cook?* This is a standard saying from individuals who don't recognize how simple and quick it can be to prepare their own meals and start eating healthier.

Start by adding one more meal at home each week. Cooking and eating healthy is like any other skill. It takes a little practice to perfect. So don't worry if you get frustrated at first. It's okay to burn the rice or overcook the vegetables.

After a couple of attempts it will become simpler and faster. Start with easy dishes. Cooking and eating healthy doesn't have to be disconcerting.

Now yes, I wish you the best in your results, and remember, everything is practical; theory without action is of no use to you.

*A big hug, your friend, Jessy!*

By the way, when you achieve your results little by little, I highly recommend you, if you want to learn about methods of losing weight, my book, "Learn to maximize your metabolism", is a book that I'm sure will help you a lot on your path to "good health".

Without further ado, you can find it in the Amazon search engine by its title or by looking for my name as: "Jessy M. Brown"... Once again I wish you success in your results!